Glutathione: Master Antioxidant and Detoxifier - Slow Aging, Improve Mental Function, & Increase Energy With This Universal Natural Drug

William McDaniel

© 2015

Disclaimer

Table of Contents

Introduction

Are you looking for a way to improve your general health and well-being, stave off the signs of aging and help boost your resistance to dread diseases at the same time?

The problem for most of us today is that life gets too busy – with the internet and smart phones, we are constantly connected. Technology has, instead of reducing our workload, increased it exponentially.

Being under constant stress and pressure makes it a lot harder to actually stick to a healthy diet and a lot simpler to reach for the nearest take out menu. As a result, lifestyle diseases such as diabetes and cardiovascular disease have become a global epidemic.

Obesity and inflammatory diseases are no longer the exception. Many Americans suffer from chronic pain every day of their lives. Many of us can be best described as the walking wounded – not well enough to be classified as vibrantly healthy but not ill enough to be considered diseased.

Being vibrantly healthy is your birthright and in this book I am going to share how you can start working towards being vibrantly healthy today.

There are tons of books out there purporting to do the same but the problem is that these recycle the same old information over and over again – eat right and exercise.

This book is different in that I will not be telling you to improve your diet or even to start exercising. There is not one magic diet plan out there that will work for everyone. You probably already know what foods you should be eating.

What I am going to do is to introduce you to an amino acid that is essential for a healthy life, one that counters the damage caused by oxidative stress and that can assist you in living a healthier life – Glutathione

Never heard of it? I am not surprised – this is one amino acid that does not get the press that it deserves, especially considering how hard it works.

In this book I will explain to you what glutathione actually is, why it works and how it works on the different body systems. We will look at whether or not you should be taking it and, if so, how much to take and what format you should be taking it in.

Depending on where you currently are health-wise, it may be difficult to even consider implementing major life changes. I know that – chronic illness or pain saps your energy and vitality to such an extent that it hard to implement major changes that will be of benefit to you.

This book is not about major changes that you have to accomplish – all that is required of you is to make one change for now. Once the Glutathione kicks in, you will have the energy and ability to make more significant changes towards a healthier lifestyle.

What Is Glutathione?

Glutathione is not one of the most complex compounds that your body produces – all it really is a combination of glycine, glutamine and cysteine. This little tripeptide does pack one massive punch though – it is essential for the health of every cell in the body and, despite the fact that it is manufactured throughout the entire body, there is a very good chance that you are not making enough of it.

And that's the rub. Your body has to have this compound in order to combat illness and in order to increase vitality but your body's ability to make the compound is impaired by the stresses of day to day living and the environmental toxins that it is exposed to.

What makes it so powerful is the Sulphur that it contains. Sulphur can be compared to tacky glue for toxins and free-radicals. These molecules attract the heavy metals and free radicals in the system and help to speed them out of your system.

Under normal circumstances, the body copes with these toxins quite well. The problem is that "normal" living today causes us to encounter a barrage of toxins. The body is simply no longer able to cope anymore.

In addition, some of us have started off with a disadvantage anyway – the genes that regulate glutathione production do not work as well as they should and so our ability to cope with toxic overload is impaired as well.

When our forebears were evolving into the form that we are familiar with today, there simply was no need to detoxify the system at the same level as what we do today – environmental toxins were just not present at such massive levels at the time.

In fact, no other generation has had to face such a preponderance of chemicals and toxicity. A couple of hundred years ago, before the industrial revolution, we still lived relatively simple lives – we had no option but to eat real food that was prepared from scratch and we had no factories belching out pollutants as they do today.

Today there are so many options when it comes to the food we eat, it is astounding – foods that our ancestors could never have dreamed of. Food full of preservatives, flavorants and colorants that simply weren't even known about back then. It is conservatively estimated that in the last seventy years alone, since the end of World War II, there are more than eighty five thousand chemical compounds that have been registered.

Put quite simply, we were not designed to cope with the huge amounts of toxins that we are now exposed to on a daily basis and, in around about half the population today, this limited ability to deal with toxins has been carried through in the genes.

When it comes to chronic illness, the body's reserves are further sapped over time. In time, glutathione production is decreased to significantly low levels, meaning that there is further toxic buildup and even more illness. It becomes a vicious cycle – as glutathione levels decrease, the levels of toxins in the body increase, making it harder for the body to function normally – eventually, the body spirals out of control and you get more and more ill.

We are not only robbed of our health but also get progressively more ill as time passes and the more ill we become, the less we have the ability to produce glutathione.

This affects every aspect of our day to day lives – even damaging the very cells that give us our energy. Not only are you more prone to develop serious illness, but you are also sapped of vital energy that would previously have given you the strength to fight back.

It is not for nothing that studies have shown that those people suffering from degenerative diseases like arthritis, Alzheimer's, Parkinson's and the like have been shown to have lower than average levels of glutathione.

Fortunately though, it is not all doom and gloom – even if you are already seriously ill and severely deficient in glutathione, you can increase your body's ability to both produce and effectively use glutathione and look forward to better health and a brighter future.

Whilst glutathione does not necessarily completely reverse the effects of some serious illnesses, it can help to prevent them progressing further and can help in the treatment of symptoms overall.

It also boosts the retention of Vitamins C and E and so has a general knock on effect when it comes to the levels of these nutrients as well. Conversely, ensuring that you get sufficient quantities of these vitamins can also help to ensure that your glutathione levels do not become depleted. These three compounds therefore act synergistically and so their action overall is improved in the presence of one another.

Glutathione and the Chronically Ill

The reason that glutathione is so important in the body is that it helps to neutralize free radicals that would otherwise cause severe problems in the body.

What Are Free Radicals?

Free radicals are more harmful to the body than any toxins that you ingest – free radicals are very unstable and react on a molecular level to disrupt cellular processes. In the process, the cells in the body are damaged and so their functions are impaired.

What is more, the free radical effect causes a chain reaction in the cells of the body so basically even a relatively small amount of free radicals in the body can cause a great deal of damage.

The damage is cumulative and if the free radicals are not dealt with decisively, their effects will become more and more damaging over time, leading to higher levels of inflammation and illness.

Anti-oxidants such as glutathione and vitamin E bind with the free radicals and so render them harmless. In order to neutralize the free radicals effectively, you need to take in more anti-oxidants. With today's lifestyle, however, that is becoming more and more difficult because the anti-oxidants that we need are found primarily in fresh fruit and vegetables.

Your standard Western diet is loaded with highly refined and processed foods, with little in the way of fresh fruit and vegetables.

Sugar is the drug of choice for many of us and it is much more lethal than heroin or cocaine and just as addictive. The more sugar and refined foods that you eat, the more you want – sugar acts on the same pleasure receptors in the brain that drugs do and so, once you are hooked, your body actually experiences symptoms of withdrawal and cravings that are every bit as powerful as a craving for drugs can be.

Worse still, the refined sugars and carbohydrates that we are so fond of have very little in terms of nutritive value and actually lead to the development of free radicals within the body. We are poisoning ourselves slowly when it comes to sugar and refined carbohydrates.

The more rubbish that we eat, the more glutathione that we need. As time goes on, the body's stores of glutathione become depleted and we are no longer able to fight the effects of the free radicals. We simply do not give the body the basic building blocks that it needs to fight illness.

This leads to chronic inflammation which, in turn leads to chronic illness.

And as if that was not bad enough, depleting your stores of glutathione leads to a weakened immune system. Your immune system needs glutathione in order to function properly.

The glutathione binds to the toxins and carries them out of the body via the waste systems.

In addition, lower levels of glutathione has been linked to increased risk of muscle damage, a reduced ability to heal quickly, loss of stamina and strength and the reduction in the ability to build new muscle.

In fact, in those diagnosed with HIV, studies have shown that the triggering of full blown AIDS can be attributed to the depletion of glutathione stores.

Glutathione is essential for the healthy functioning of the immune system because it boosts the activation of T-Cells in the blood and helps to maintain a healthy balance between the various T-Cells.

It has been found that it not even necessary to completely deplete the glutathione levels to really decrease the action of the immune system dramatically. Decreasing the levels to even 40% of what they should be – easy enough to do in today's environment – can completely reduce the body's ability to activate T-Cells, meaning that you will be even more prone to developing infections and illnesses.

Should You Be Supplementing Your Glutathione Intake?

The answer to this question, for just about everyone, is a resounding yes. The amounts that you need will depend on what state you are in now health-wise, how many fresh fruits and vegetables you eat and how many toxins that you are exposed to– like if you need to take medication - on a day to day basis.

In this chapter we will deal with these three issues.

Glutathione is generally considered safe for use in adults and it is hard to overdose on it since the body will simply excrete what it does not use.

That said, there are some contraindications – if you are pregnant or asthmatic, or if you have cancer it is better not to supplement it but to boost the levels naturally by eating more fruit and vegetables.

How Healthy Are You?

If you are reading this book, there is a good chance that you are not in the best shape health-wise. If you are battling ill health or have been chronically ill for some time, there is a better than average chance that your glutathione levels are lower than they should be.

Try doing a simple experiment to see whether or not you need to increase the glutathione levels that your body produces – there is no need for expensive blood tests – just try including more fresh vegetables today and every day for a week.

If you find that you are starting to feel better with this, it is a good bet that you are low when it comes to glutathione production.

How Many Fresh Fruits And Vegetables Do You Eat?

I said that I was not going to lecture you about your diet and I did mean it. However, if you are not eating enough fresh produce, there is a really good chance that you are not giving your body the nutrients that it needs in order to produce glutathione.

The recommended daily allowance when it comes to fresh fruit and vegetables is 5-9 servings a day. This is not as hard to achieve as is sounds – one serving can be as little as half a cup of frozen vegetables or one medium-sized piece of fruit.

How Many Toxins You Are Exposed To

If you live in a city where environmental pollutants are high; if you are taking medication on a daily basis or if you are eating a lot of added sugar, there is a better than average chance that your glutathione levels are too low.

If you have been exposed to heavy metals in any way or feel that you may be in danger of being exposed to heavy metals, increasing your glutathione production should be attempted. The glutathione chelates these heavy metals. What this basically means is that it binds itself to these heavy metals so that they are excreted with the body's waste.

When it comes to environmental pollutants, it is better to err on the side of caution – most people are taking in a lot more toxins than they realize – they can be present in the food that we eat, the water that we drink and the air that we breathe. Many toxins are present in the products that we apply to our skins on a daily basis and they are there legally.

When Not to Take A Glutathione Supplement

Glutathione has not been proven safe to use during pregnancy so it is wiser not to supplement it whilst pregnant. As a pregnant woman, you really do need to be more careful when it comes to what food you eat anyway – despite the cravings. If you are pregnant, I would look at boosting your intake through your diet – by providing your body with the precursors that it needs to produce enough glutathione. As long as it has enough basic ingredients, it can make enough glutathione on its own without the need for supplementation.

It is also not a good idea to supplement glutathione if you have asthma because it can aggravate some of the symptoms. It may seem crazy, but N-Acetyl-Cysteine can actually be helpful in treating some of the symptoms of asthma. Again, try boosting your levels through diet and making sure that you get enough of the precursors without actually supplementing glutathione itself.

If you have been diagnosed with cancer, it is advisable not to take glutathione as it is needed by all cells, not just the healthy ones and can actually boost the production of cancerous cells as well as healthy ones. In general, when it comes to cancer, following a more simple approach to your diet and eating more "real" food is bound to be an effective way to help you to deal with the symptoms of the cancer and the side effects of the treatment as well.

So, in general, if you want to boost your health and are not pregnant or asthmatic, you can safely supplement your natural glutathione levels.

They say that aging isn't for wimps and it is generally accepted that our bodies will decline as we age. In truth though, there is nothing natural about becoming more and more ill as we get older and that is really great news.

What this means is that you can actually prevent the ravages of aging to a large extent. In ancient times, the average person died at the ripe old age of 28. Today, that is not even considered middle-aged anymore. More and more people are living into their 80's and 90's - the average maximum age for a person living in a developed country is 84 now.

What that shows us is that as we learn more and more about what makes our body tick and using that knowledge, we are living and remaining active for longer and longer – the body is absolutely amazing and has the ability to enable us to stay "young" for longer now. Although it may not always seem like it, the body is very good at regulating itself and imbalances or disease are very often symptoms of nutrient deficiencies than natural developments. It all depends on what support we give our bodies.

So, if our bodies are so amazing, why are so many of us chronically ill? The simple truth is that we are simply overwhelming our body's natural defense mechanisms and setting ourselves up to develop illness and disease – one cheeseburger and coke at a time.

For starters, our bodies are exposed to a lot of environmental toxins. Add in stress and bad eating habits and you have a recipe for disaster as your body gets less of the nutrients that it needs in order to cope and ever-increasing loads of stressors are added.

As we get older, the body has little choice but to surrender and admit that it is completely overwhelmed and so the signs of aging start to show. We have simply begun to

accept this as a natural phenomenon rather than what it is –
our body's cry for help.

What is interesting is that studies have shown a direct
correlation between the levels of glutathione in the body
and overall health and vitality and that, there is a definite
correlation between levels of glutathione in the body and
longevity.

Science tells us that glutathione production slows down as
we age but, again, this does not seem like a natural
phenomenon as levels in people who lived active and
healthy lives in old age matched those of healthy people in
their thirties and forties.

Although the compound was actually discovered over a
hundred years ago, serious research only really began in
the 1920's. At the time it was discovered that glutathione
was very effective at improving the health of the lens of
the eye and that it could help prevent the formation of

cataracts as well - most of the research centered around using it to prevent macular degeneration.

Since then, more studies have been conducted on the anti-aging benefits of glutathione and it has been found that this is where this compound really thrives. It literally acts as a sponge to mop up free radicals in the body and to completely neutralize them.

What Makes Free Radicals So Dangerous?

To answer that question, we need to do a quick review of high school chemistry. Remember those lessons about atoms?

Every atom has a number of protons, neutrons and electrons that surround it. The electrons are paired with the protons and this forms your molecule. Where there is a strong and balanced bond, you get a very stable molecule that will basically not react with anything.

When the bond is weak or there is an unbalanced number of protons and electrons, the molecule will try to re-establish balance by either drawing in or shedding electrons or sharing electrons with an adjacent molecule.

A free radical then is simply a molecule that tries to rebalance itself by taking electrons from adjacent cells. The problem is that this then causes an imbalance in those molecules and they, in turn, have to scavenge for molecules from other cells and so a chain reaction is begun, leaving a wake of damaged cells behind.

Initially, the body is able to cope with this damage and carry on as normal. As you get older, however, the damage accumulates and you start to see the effects of degeneration of the cells.

Antioxidants are effective at reducing the levels of free radicals because they are very stable molecules – when they bond with the free radicals, it has little effect on their stability. The free radicals thus get the electrons that they need and the chain reaction is stopped dead in its tracks.

This has a direct effect in helping the body fight the degenerative effects of aging because it prevents the cells from becoming damaged in the first place.

Naturally though, you need to have a higher level of antioxidants than free radicals in your system in order to get positive effects.

Glutathione is the most effective antioxidant that the body has at its disposal and the one with the biggest benefit in terms of stopping degeneration due to aging.

Studies have shown that people with degenerative diseases such as arthritis typically have very low levels of glutathione in their systems and that these people were more likely to die at a younger age. Conversely, those that lived the longest – those in the age group 80-95 – typically had high levels of glutathione in their systems.

As glutathione is required by every cell in the body, the effects of a deficiency are quite widespread – you will literally see these effects from head to toe.

Glutathione has long been used as a treatment to whiten skin but its effects are a lot more profound than that – it can help to reduce the appearance of your skin in general and prevent the formation of fine lines and wrinkles. It also helps to reduce the appearance of age spots. Your skin looks younger and is healthier in general.

The jury is thus quite firmly in on this one – if you want to live a longer and healthier life, and, at the same time, look younger, you need to increase your levels of glutathione.

Get Back Your Energy And Vitality

When it comes to the cells in your body, you need four basic things in order to keep them healthy and alive – oxygen, water, glutathione and glucose.

These things are necessary in order for your cells to produce energy. Think of them as you would the battery in your mobile phone – without the battery, you phone is dead. The same applies to your cells.

Your body can run on less than optimal levels of these compounds but again, it is just like your mobile phone – as the battery gets weaker, the phone does not perform as well. The weaker the battery, the weaker the signal it is able to send out and, eventually, your phone dies. Your body is exactly the same.

When your body has the right level of nutrients, it is like when you have just charged your phone – it works at optimal capacity.

The so-called mitochondrial disorders are also becoming rife now. Conditions like fibromyalgia, lupus and chronic fatigue arise when there has been damage to the mitochondria in your cells.

The mitochondria are essentially the cell's batteries and they are also susceptible to damage from free radicals.

Glutathione not only repairs this damage but it helps to prevent further damage being done. This, in turn, will help to restore energy production at a cellular level.

Not only will your cells have the energy that they need to function, but there will be extra energy left over for you to use as well.

Reduce Inflammation

Inflammation is one of the body's natural defense mechanisms and it is intended to prevent further damage and promote healing. It is basically a sign that your body is dealing with an infection or injury and it is your body's attempt to get rid of whatever has triggered the response.

Inflammation is thus a biological necessity. Without it, wounds would not heal and the body would not be able to fight off disease. So basically, we don't want to cut out inflammation completely. There is a point, however, when you can get too much of a good thing and your inflammatory response is a prime example of that.

Inflammation is, however, meant to be a short-term response. If the inflammation is not removed for a prolonged period, the body's healing processes are hampered rather than aided. Long-term inflammation is extremely damaging to your body and predisposes you to develop the so-called lifestyle disease. In these cases, the inflammatory response is triggered even when it is not necessary and causes further inflammation in the body. It is as if your body is at red alert all the time.

The body basically starts attacking the healthy tissue as well. More prostaglandins are produced and this, in turn, causes more pain and swelling. The inflammatory response is triggered again and a vicious cycle begins as a result.

Because there are too many messengers floating around your blood stream, inflammation becomes a system-wide problem and more and more healthy tissues and cells are affected and the body becomes less and less able to heal itself.

Glutathione fights inflammation in two ways – first of all, it protects the cells from free radical damage. Secondly, it helps to stop the inflammatory cascade in its tracks and this is what prevents further damage due to inflammation, especially in people who have an overactive inflammatory response.

The problem when it comes to the inflammatory response is that this response can cascade out of control. It is very difficult to stop this cascade when it happens initially but glutathione can do just that.

Also, by removing harmful toxins from our systems, the glutathione can help to prevent the inflammatory response in the first place.

You can further boost this anti-inflammatory action by getting enough Omega-3 fatty acids. Omega-3 fatty acids assist the body in fighting inflammation and, much like fruit and vegetables, most of us do not get enough of it.

You can get enough by eating oily fish like salmon twice a week or through taking a supplement. Do be careful not to supplement Omega-6 fatty acids if you are already suffering from inflammation. Many supplements do contain both but most of us actually get too many Omega-6 fatty acids from our diets anyway.

Omega-6 fatty acids are important as well but we need 10 times as much Omega-3's as we do Omega-6's. When you have too many Omega-6 fatty acids in your body, they will stimulate the production of prostaglandins and consequently increase the inflammation in your body.

Omega-6's are available in high quantities in vegetable oils and that is why most of us have such high levels in our bloodstream.

In addition to Omega-6's, another problem with our Western diet is that it usually includes a lot of trans-fats. These are even worse for you when it comes to inflammation and should be avoided as far as possible.

Trans-fats are usually formed when fats are heated to high levels. What happens is that the fats are chemically transformed and they become more volatile and more prone to oxidation.

Glutathione and Diabetes

Type II or adult-onset diabetes develops as a result of one of a couple of different conditions. If the pancreas fails to produce enough insulin, or the cells of the body become insulin resistant, Diabetes develops.

The scary thing is that adult-onset diabetes accounts for about 9 out 10 cases. Considering that this is a disease that can be prevented, this stat is even more alarming.

Basically the cells in the body do not get enough insulin in order to convert the glucose in our food into energy. Excess glucose is then taken to the liver and converted into fat – to be stored there or in other parts of our bodies.

The consequences of diabetes are dire – sufferers are at risk of developing renal failure and a number of other serious health complications.

Studies have shown that the glutathione level in diabetics is a lot lower than that the norm.

Diabetes actually saps the body's ability to produce glutathione by actually reducing the amount of glycine and cysteine in the body.

If the diabetes is uncontrolled, glutathione levels are usually always severely restricted leading to even more free radical damage and further damage. The mitochondria of the cells become damaged and energy levels plummet even further.

It is extremely important that people with diabetes do supplement their diets with either reduced glutathione or the precursors to it. Doing so can assist in cellular repair and the prevention of further damage.

Symptoms that may mean you have diabetes include:

If you find that you have gained or lost a good deal of weight for no good reason;

If you find that you have an increased need to urinate;

If you find that you are constantly thirsty;

If you find that your vision has become impaired.

This is not an exhaustive list of symptoms but these are the primary indicators that you may be either diabetic or pre-diabetic. If you have a history of diabetes in your family, it is important to watch out for these symptoms.

If you are careful enough and you catch it early enough, your symptoms need never develop into full blown diabetes and you will be able to control them through diet alone.

The primary concern when it comes to diet is, strangely enough, not just monitoring the sugar that you eat – fat also plays a significant role here. You do need to be careful if you are buying "diabetic" friendly products because they will often improve the flavor by adding more fat – let's face it, fat and sugar make food taste really good so most diet foods will contain one or the other.

It is better to steer clear of artificially sweetened foods and drinks because these do not fool the body anyway – it is not sated by these foods and you will find that you still crave sugar. Where possible, cut sugar out completely.

Glutathione and Your Liver

Your liver is one of the few organs that is capable of regenerating itself. It has amazing regenerative properties and can take quite a good beating but, eventually, the effects of an unhealthy lifestyle will start to show in decreased liver function.

The liver is the primary organ that your body needs to remove toxins from the system and glutathione is essential for the proper functioning of the liver.

Glutathione acts as an antioxidant in the liver, protecting it from oxidative damage and improving liver regeneration. It is also essential to assist the liver in removing toxins and heavy metals from your system.

Getting enough glutathione for your liver is important when it comes to decreasing the chances of you developing liver disease – once serious liver damage has set in, it is difficult, if not impossible, to reverse.

If you have already developed a form of liver disease, you can go a long way towards halting the progression of the disease as whole by boosting your intake of glutathione.

You can boost the production of glutathione in the liver and further support liver health by taking a Milk Thistle supplement on a daily basis. I have gone into this in more detail further on in the book but you should be taking 100mg of Milk Thistle with 80% Sylmarin content on a daily basis to support healthy liver function.

This becomes especially important if you take medication of any sort or if you drink alcohol on a day to day basis. It is especially important if you take a few different medications daily – even if your doctor has prescribed your medications and you need to take them for health reasons, they are still synthetic chemicals that may leave behind a toxic residue and this needs to be scrubbed out of the system.

Milk thistle can assist with this.

As a bonus, Milk Thistle can help you to lose weight by helping to clear out your gut.

Glutathione And Your Cognitive Health

Because of the antioxidant effect of glutathione, it has tremendous benefits when it comes to cognitive health and the prevention of diseases such as Alzheimer's and Parkinson's Diseases.

In one study it was found that supplementation with N-Acetyl-Cysteine could arrest the further deterioration of elderly patients showing the early signs of dementia.

Glutathione has proven especially helpful in treating neurological diseases. It has proven especially promising in trials to treat Parkinson's disease, helping to not only halt the progress of the disease itself but also in restoring some normal function to sufferers. In these trials, the glutathione was given intravenously so it is not expected that home users would achieve the same sort of results but the study overall is encouraging.

Improvement in the patients was marked – with significant results manifesting in just a month of treatment – in some cases improvement in the symptoms of Parkinson's disease was as much as 42%.

This also points to promising results in terms of the prevention of cognitive deterioration as well.

Glutathione is not only good for the elderly when it comes to memory though – it can assist anyone in helping improve the memory.

The effects of stress and oxidative damage on the brain should not be underestimated and they can be quite severe, leading to a decrease in the ability of the brain to retain facts and sometimes even the ability to process information.

By helping the body to deal with the oxidative stress and by increasing the amount of energy available as a whole, glutathione has proven to be a useful ally in the fight against stress.

Combine your increased uptake of glutathione with sufficient levels of the B Vitamins and you have a recipe for success.

Again, the reduction in cognitive function is not a natural and unavoidable progression but rather a symptom of an underlying nutrient deficiency.

It is also important when fighting memory loss and cognitive disease that you get enough essential fatty acids. This means eating oily fish at least twice a week. If, like me, you do not like fish, a high quality fish oil supplement, should be taken on a daily basis.

Some people say that flaxseed is a suitable substitute but this is not the case – flaxseed does contain essential fatty acids but not in a form that your body can actually use.

As mentioned in the earlier chapters, choosing a glutathione supplement needs to be approached with care because glutathione itself will not survive the digestive process. Get the wrong type of glutathione and all you are doing, at best, is wasting your money – if you cannot find reduced glutathione, you will need to consider either having intravenous supplementation or increasing your intake of the precursors.

Intravenous Supplementation

This has proven to be one of the most effective ways to administer glutathione but it can be a costly exercise as the treatment needs to be administered in a clinic. This can also prove quite inconvenient at the same time.

If you are chronically ill and really battling with pain, I advise taking a glutathione supplement for at least three months to give you a boost and then look at ways to incorporate it more naturally into your diet.

Foods That Help Your Body Produce The Glutathione That It Needs

If you are at all concerned that you might be taking too much of the supplement or if you are not keen on adding another supplement to your daily list, you can naturally increase the body's production of glutathione by providing it with the nutrients that it needs to product it.

Supplement Your Diet With Whey Protein

If you are not lactose intolerant and if you can find bioactive whey powder, you might consider taking a whey protein powder as whey is a really good source of cysteine and amino acids that are essential for glutathione production.

Try, as far as possible, to get one that is as organic as possible.

Increasing Output Through Exercise

If you feel up to it, you can start introducing exercise into your daily life as this boosts the levels of glutathione in the body. Aim for half an hour of aerobic exercise – i.e. increasing your heart rate – on a daily basis and add in about half an hour of strength training every alternate day or so.

Again, I promised that I would not lecture on the benefits of exercise so only try to exercise when you start to feel better.

If you have not exercised in a while, or you are unfit, it is better to start off slowly and to progress as you feel fitter.

Aim to walk around the block initially and gradually increase the time spent exercising until you have managed to get the recommended amounts. You want to raise your heart rate enough so that you are a little out of breath but not so much that you are not able to carry a conversation. (No puffing and wheezing up the hill then!)

Exercise does not necessarily mean that you have to stand on the treadmill. Choose something that you actually enjoy doing in order to increase the chances that you will be able to maintain the pace.

On the whole, if exercise becomes too much of a chore, you are not going to be able to keep it up so do not be too hard on yourself, at least when you are starting out.

If possible, find someone who is supportive and get them to go with you. Try and find someone who is around the same level of fitness that you are and you can both encourage each other to succeed. It is important to get someone who is supportive and not a tyrant – I once signed up for gym and went with my cousin and I hated every minute of it because he was a lot fitter and kept on "encouraging" me. Then he wanted to get to the gym at 4:30 in the morning and I decided that enough was enough – I had made two cardinal mistakes – I was forcing myself to go even though I hated it and it had really become a chore.

I realized that I could have a lot more fun taking dance classes or long walks and so that became my "gym".

Increase Levels Through Supplementation

Saying that you can take a glutathione supplement is a little bit of a misnomer because a pure glutathione supplement by itself would not survive the digestive process. If taking it a supplement form, you need to ensure that it is reduced glutathione or you are really just wasting your money. That said, it can be safely given intravenously or in the form of a gas. Neither is particularly convenient for home users so what you can do instead is to provide the body with the right building blocks so that it can make more of its own glutathione.

At the end of the day, there is some debate as to whether or not taking too much of one particular antioxidant is, in fact, helpful so if you are still relatively healthy, I would advise increasing the levels of glutathione supporting nutrients so that your body can decide how much it needs to produce.

These nutrients include:

N-acetyl-cysteine: This supplement has been used to great effect in the treatment of respiratory tract disorders such as lung disease and asthma. It is also a standard treatment for the treatment of an overdose of Tylenol. It also helps to prevent renal damage as a result of the use of chemical dyes for x-ray purposes.

Alpha lipoic acid: The body requires this in its basic form for energy production, the control of blood sugar, detoxification and cognitive function in addition to using it as a building block for glutathione. This is another of the nutrients that the body can produce itself but is one that we are very often short of.

Vitamins B6, B12 and Folate: When it comes to glutathione production, these are vital. Methylation is one of the most important functions in the body as a whole. Look for folate in the form of 5 methyltetrahydrofolate; B6 in the form of P5P and B12 listed as methylcobalamin. If you are under a great deal of stress, it is especially important to supplement the B Vitamins as the body's stores are more quickly depleted when the body during these times.

Selenium: Selenium is an important nutrient in its own right but is also essential for boosting the production of glutathione. With Selenium, it is important to stick to the recommended daily allowance of a maximum of 200 mcg and not to exceed this as excess levels in the body will be stored and can build to toxic levels. If you love Brazil nuts and eat them just about every day, skip Selenium in supplement form as Brazil nuts contain a lot of Selenium.

Antioxidants such as Vitamin C and E: These are important to help the body to actively use the glutathione and work to help prevent the depletion and boost the action of the glutathione. It should be remembered that Vitamin E is

Milk Thistle: Long known for helping repair liver damage and to help detoxify the body, milk thistle can also help boost the levels of glutathione produced. The active ingredient, Silymarin has been shown to boost the levels of glutathione in the liver by 35% in human trials.

L Glutamine: When used in conjunction with N-Acetyl-Cysteine, L- Glutamine supplementation has been proven to restore glutathione stores. It can also help to reduce the digestive upsets caused by some chemotherapy drugs and to further enhance the functioning of the immune system and ability to heal in individuals who have undergone radiation treatment, bone marrow transplants and surgery. It helps reduce the rate of infection in such cases.

Quantities Necessary To Boost Glutathione Levels

Significantly

In order to maintain good glutathione levels, you need to take a general multi-vitamin supplement. Choose a good quality, high potency supplement that contains as few fillers and additives as possible. You need to ensure that you take the following vitamins and minerals on a daily basis in the quantities recommended:

1000 mg of Vitamin C (Vitamin C is water-soluble so excess amounts will be flushed out of the system).

Vitamin E Succinate – 400 IU (Vitamin E is fat-soluble so do not exceed this dosage or it can build up to toxic levels).

Selenium 100-200 mcg (You need to be careful with Selenium as it can build up to toxic levels in the tissues so do not exceed this dosage).

Beta-carotene – 10,000 -20,000 IU (Again, whilst this is a fairly safe compound, do not exceed this dosage).

Vitamin A – 2500 IU (Vitamin A is fat soluble and so do not exceed this dosage or it can build up to toxic levels)

It is a good idea to also take the following additional nutrients, over and above your vitamin and mineral supplement, on a daily basis in order to maintain healthy levels of glutathione production – for the sake of convenience, we will assume that you are able to find all of the following ingredients in a single capsule form – this makes it easier to understand the dosage guidelines laid out underneath:

350 mg of N-Acetyl Cysteine

75 mg of Alpha – Lipoic acid

300 mg of L- Glutamine

100 mg of Milk Thistle - ensuring that you get one that has at least 80% silymarin content.

The following guidelines with regards to dosage will assist when treating the conditions listed (Just remember that these dosages only apply to the additional nutrients and not the general vitamin and mineral supplement):

1 capsule taken in the morning for people wishing to improve their general good health.

Between 2 and four capsules on a daily basis, divided into equal doses over breakfast and lunch for those suffering from liver complaints.

Between 2 and four capsules on a daily basis, divided into equal doses over breakfast and lunch for those suffering from renal illnesses.

1 or 2 capsules a day after breakfast for those taking acetaminophen or drinking alcohol on a regular basis.

1 or 2 capsules a day after breakfast for those taking multiple prescription drugs on a daily basis.

Between 3 and 4 capsules on a daily basis, divided into equal doses over breakfast and lunch for those diagnosed with HIV.

2 capsules daily with breakfast to help get rid of mucus in those who have bronchitis.

2 capsules daily – one after breakfast and one after lunch to help improve the body's tolerance to glucose in those who have diabetes.

4 capsules daily – two after breakfast and two after lunch in those who have Parkinson's Disease, Multiple Sclerosis or Amytrophic Lateral Sclerosis.

Between 1 and 4 capsules a day – divided over breakfast and lunch – to help deal with exposure to heavy metals – the final dosage will depend on how bad the exposure has been.

2 capsules per day to help prevent further cataracts forming.

2 capsules per day to help reverse polycystic ovarian disease.

2-4 capsules a day – divided over breakfast and lunch – to treat early stage Alzheimer's Disease and dementia.

I do find that Milk Thistle does make me a bit nauseous when I supplement it so if you are finding that the regimen above leaves you feeling nauseous, separate out the Milk Thistle from your supplementation and take it last thing at night before you go to bed. That way you will be asleep and digestive upsets will be kept to a minimum.

Conclusion

Thank you for downloading this book.

I hope that you have learned a lot about the benefits of glutathione and how you can boost your own levels of this vital compound.

I also hope that this is really helpful to you when it comes to combatting pain and illness – there really is no reason why we should not all be healthy and feel well every single day and if I have helped just one person achieve a higher level of wellness, I will consider the time taken to write this book very well spent indeed.

Glutathione is one of the building blocks of good health and longevity and studies have shown that there is a direct link between low levels of glutathione and high levels of disease and degeneration linked to aging and inflammation. Keep yourself healthy and active into your twilight years by ensuring that your body has adequate levels of this nutrient.

I would like to ask one thing of you before you leave – I would really appreciate feedback from you and I would love to learn whether or not this book has helped you. When you have a moment, please review this book on Amazon for me and, if you have started seeing the benefits of glutathione in your own life, please drop me a line.

Your feedback would be most appreciated!

Here's to a happy, healthy and long life.

www.ingramcontent.com/pod-product-compliance
Lightning Source LLC
Chambersburg PA
CBHW070323290526
45791CB00003B/1236